Domingos Diletieri Carvalho

Study of the use of anesthetics

Domingos Diletieri Carvalho

Study of the use of anesthetics

Adverse Drug Reactions

ScienciaScripts

This book is a translation from the original published under ISBN 978-613-9-61655-8.

Publisher:
Sciencia Scripts
is a trademark of
Dodo Books Indian Ocean Ltd. and OmniScriptum S.R.L publishing group

120 High Road, East Finchley, London, N2 9ED, United Kingdom
Str. Armeneasca 28/1, office 1, Chisinau MD-2012, Republic of Moldova, Europe
Printed at: see last page
ISBN: 978-620-7-88643-2

Table of contents:

Chapter 1

1. INTRODUCTION

Pain is a complex sensory quality, often unrelated to the degree of tissue damage. Pain, according to the International Association for the Study of Pain (AIED), is defined as an unpleasant emotional sensation and experience associated with actual or potential tissue damage (ROCHA, 2002).

The effort to suppress pain caused by surgical procedures through the use of drugs dates back to antiquity, including the oral administration of ethanol and opiates. The first scientific demonstration of drug-induced anesthesia during surgery was made in 1846 in Boston, when William Morton used diethyl ether. A year later, chloroform was introduced by James Simpson in Scotland. These first steps were followed 20 years later by the successful demonstration of the anesthetic properties of nitrous oxide, which had first been suggested by Sir Humphry Davy in the 1790s. Modern anesthesia dates back to the 1930s, when thiopental, an intravenous barbiturate, was introduced. A decade later, curare was used in anesthesia to achieve skeletal muscle relaxation. The first modern halogenated hydrocarbon, halothane, was introduced as an inhaled anesthetic in 1956 and soon became the standard of comparison for new inhaled anesthetic drugs (KATZUNG, 2003).

The history of the application of local anesthetics (LA) via the spinal route is quite old, and its use was first documented by Bier in 1899. In 1940, Lemmon introduced the idea of continuous infusion of anesthetic and, in 1948, Lofgren presented his thesis defending the use of spinal lidocaine, which began the application of this substance for surgical procedures (ROCHA, 2002).

Technological advances in healthcare have made it possible to perform less invasive surgical procedures with the aim of reducing the incidence of complications, length of stay and hospital costs (SANTOS, 2006).

Data from a review of mortality associated with anesthetic-surgical procedures shows a decrease in mortality over the last 50 years. Some authors, however, believe that the incidence of adverse events is directly related to morbidity factors intrinsic to patients (CICARELLI, 2005).

Pharmacoepidemiology "is a field of study that forms a bridge between pharmacology, therapeutics, epidemiology and statistics. It is the application of epidemiological reasoning and methods to the study of the effects, both beneficial and adverse (pharmacovigilance), and the use of medicines in the population". It is an area of great social importance, given its potential to contribute to reducing health expenditure, directly, by rationalizing the use of medicines and, indirectly, by reducing iatrogenic problems (COELHO; ARRAIS, 1999).

The general objective of this work was to study the use of general and local anesthetics in patients assisted by a public hospital. The specific objectives were: to detect the prevalence of anaesthetic use in hospitalized patients; to study all forms of anaesthetic use, comparing the data found with the scientific literature; to detect possible adverse reactions or known and unknown drug interactions among patients using this class of drug; to monitor the appearance of the main known adverse reactions to this class of drug; to record and report possible adverse reactions presented by patients using anaesthetics.

Chapter 2

2. LITERATURE REVIEW

2.1 Pharmacovigilance

Medicines have become an important therapeutic tool in the treatment and prophylaxis of many illnesses, and are responsible for improving people's quality of life. For pharmacotherapy to be successful and produce the expected results, the drug must be used for the appropriate clinical conditions, prescribed in the appropriate pharmaceutical form, doses and duration of treatment, and the prescribed therapeutic regimen must be adhered to (Marin *et al.*, 2003). However, there is an imminent risk of adverse reactions.

Unexpected events, not foreseeable in clinical studies, which can lead to serious public health problems if not identified early.

The introduction of a growing number of drugs due to the evolution of the pharmaceutical industry and the difficulty of detecting adverse effects during clinical trials are elements that reaffirm the importance of pharmacovigilance (NISHIYAMA, 2002).

In the Dictionary of Epidemiology, "post-marketing surveillance of medicines" is the "procedure set in motion after the registration of a new drug has been authorized; designed to seek information on the actual use of the drug for a given indication, as well as on the appearance of undesirable effects. Method for the epidemiological study of adverse drug reactions" (GOMES, 2001).

In this context, once a new drug has been developed, it is necessary to develop it.

pre-clinical studies were carried out to investigate its pharmacological and toxicological activities *in vitro* and in animals. Subsequently, with the pre-clinical approval of the new drug, phase I trials are carried out on healthy volunteers to investigate safety and pharmacokinetics, phase II clinical trials are carried out on patients to study efficacy and safety in comparison with other known drugs and, finally, phase III randomized controlled clinical trials are carried out to measure the safety and efficacy of the drug on a probabilistic sample of the population. Depending on the results of the tests on human beings, the drug can then be marketed (GOMES, 2001).

However, even randomized controlled clinical trials have certain safety limitations inherent in their experimental design. For example, due to the number of individuals studied, rare effects may not be detected and, due to the length of the trial, effects resulting from prolonged use of the drug may not be revealed. It is therefore assumed that phase IV studies, pharmacovigilance or post-marketing surveillance are synonyms referring to the same process of detecting, monitoring and controlling problems arising from the already legally authorized and widespread use of medicines (GOMES, 2001). In addition, pharmacovigilance can be an important tool for promoting a cultural change that fosters a more careful perception of the use of medicines among health professionals and the population in general. Its exercise also stimulates greater concern with the teaching of Clinical Pharmacology and Pharmacoepidemiology in training courses in the health area, as well as in continuing education programs (COELHO, 1998).

In order to identify and quantify Adverse Drug Reactions, Pharmacovigilance has been implemented in Brazil through the voluntary notification system - which consists of collecting and communicating unwanted and manifested reactions after the use of a drug - by the National Health Surveillance Agency (Anvisa), with the training program for the creation of State Pharmacovigilance Systems throughout the country (ANVISA, 2004).

Brazil's interest in carrying out pharmacovigilance studies arose in the 1960s with the tragedy that haunted the whole world when it caused Phocomelia Syndrome, a deformation of the limbs of fetuses whose mothers took the drug thalidomide, indicated to combat seasickness, during pregnancy. On the one hand, thalidomide caused hundreds of children to be born without arms and legs, but on the other hand, it made health authorities around the world aware of the need to monitor the effects of commercialized drugs. Now, Brazil is starting to correct the mismatches and a well-structured program has been created for the sector, with the creation of the National Health Surveillance Agency (Anvisa), inaugurated in 1999, in which various groups of professionals, mainly pharmacists, are striving to develop pharmacovigilance, actively participating in the program through voluntary notifications (PRANDO, 2004).

2.2 *Adverse Drug Reactions*

Adverse Drug Reaction (ADR), defined as *any harmful or undesirable effect that occurs after the administration of doses normally used in humans for prophylaxis, diagnosis or treatment of an illness* (World Health Organization, 1972), has been the subject of numerous concerns. Although the aim of pharmacological therapy is to produce a cure without harming the patient, ADRs are one of the most common and most important problems in medical practice (Nishiyama, 2002).

The systematic study of ADRs, or pharmacovigilance, is aimed at detecting, evaluating, understanding and preventing the risks of adverse drug effects, and its research tools can be clinical, epidemiological, experimental or diagnostic. This knowledge is important so that a drug can be used rationally, promoting a therapy that is better suited to patients' needs and avoiding unnecessary risks. Many adverse drug effects are rare, and their toxicity is not predictable through animal experiments or controlled clinical trials. Therefore, the main objective of monitoring adverse reactions is to define, as quickly as possible, a drug's ability to produce undesirable effects (WHO, 1969).

Adverse drug reactions represent a considerable part of medical costs. It is estimated that between 3% and 8% of admissions to Internal Medicine wards are related to ADRs (EINARSON, 1993; HALLAS, et al, 1992). However, in the different medical specialties and depending on how ADRs are analyzed, the frequency of ADRs as a cause of hospital admission can vary from 3% to 40% (EINARSON, 1993). Recently, several studies have highlighted the clinical and/or economic importance of systematic studies on ADRs. All known information on ADR as a cause of hospitalization comes from countries with demographic, social and economic characteristics.

organization of health systems different from   the Brazilian reality (PFAFFENBACH, 2002).

In order to minimize the risks of ADRs and the costs of using medicines, they must be used rationally. Rational use implies certain premises that clinicians must incorporate into their usual practice. These premises are: patients should receive the most appropriate pharmacological treatment, i.e. with the minimum effective dose and for the correct length of time; it is necessary to be certain of the diagnosis and to understand the pathophysiology of the disease; it is necessary to understand the pharmacology of the available pharmacotherapeutic alternatives; it is necessary to establish targets for evaluating the efficacy and safety of the treatment, and to be willing to change the established therapy when it proves to be ineffective or toxic (PFAFFENBACH, 2002).

2.3 Pharmacoepidemiology

The use of medicines is defined by the WHO as "the marketing, distribution, prescription and use of medicines in a society, with special emphasis on the resulting medical, social and economic consequences" (WHO, 1977).

The so-called Medicines Utilization Studies (MUS) are those which, regardless of their method, objective or scope, aim to shed light on these aspects. They offer us a general view or a particular view of the use of medicines in a given society (GOMES, 2001).

The effective use of medicines is not without risks. Adverse drug reactions can affect both individuals and entire groups of vulnerable patients, with major or minor consequences that can lead to death (CASTRO, 2001).

The usefulness of applying epidemiology to the use of medicines can be thought of in two different ways: in the pre- and post-marketing periods of a new drug. The pre-marketing period is characterized by experimental research - clinical trials, the last phase of testing a drug, in which knowledge is sought about its efficacy and an assessment of its safety (GOMES, 2001).

In the 1990s, several Medicines Information Centers (MICs) were set up in Brazil. Their working characteristics make it possible to document how the population and professionals are using medicines and the possible occurrence of adverse reactions to them. These data are important elements for pharmacovigilance and studies into the use of medicines, both of which are the subject of pharmacoepidemiology. In addition, the bringing together of professionals with complementary knowledge - doctors, epidemiologists, statisticians, among others - necessary for the CIM, contributes significantly to the emergence of groups interested in carrying out pharmacoepidemiological studies. The fact that these centers are located in various regions of the country is especially conducive to the creation of a National Pharmacovigilance System (CASTRO, 1999).

The current state of research and teaching in pharmacoepidemiology in Brazil allows us to affirm that this area of knowledge will soon be consolidated in Brazil, bearing fruit in fundamental public health actions, such as the implementation of the National Pharmacovigilance System and the dissemination of informed therapy, thus making an important contribution to the realization of an essential practice for the health and quality of life of the population: the rational and safe use of medicines (CASTRO, 2001).

2.4 Drug-related problems

The concept of Drug-Related Problems (DRPs) is defined in the Second Granada Consensus as: health problems, understood as negative clinical results derived from pharmacological treatment which, produced by various causes, result in the desired therapeutic objective not being achieved or the appearance of undesirable effects (MACHUCA et al, 2004).

Thus, a DRP is a clinical outcome variable, a failure of pharmacological treatment that leads to the onset of a health problem, poor disease control or some unwanted effect. These DRPs can be of three types: related to the patient's need for medication, its effectiveness or its safety. The Second Granada Consensus establishes a classification of DRPs into six categories, which in turn are subdivided into three subcategories (Table 01).

Table 01 - Classification of Drug-Related Problems recommended by the Second Granada Consensus.

PRM classification	Categories
Need	**PRM 1:** The patient has a health problem because they are not using the pharmacotherapy they need; **PRM 2:** The patient has a health problem as a result of using a medicine they don't need;

Effectiveness	**PRM3 :** Patient presents a health problem due to a non-quantitative ineffectiveness of pharmacotherapy; **PRM4 :** Patient presents a health problem due to a quantitative ineffectiveness of pharmacotherapy;
Security	**PRM5 :** Patient presents a health problem due to a non-quantitative insecurity of a medicine; **PRM6 :** Patient presents a health problem due to a quantitative insecurity of a drug.
Source: MACHUCA, M; FERNÁNDEZ-LLIMÓS, F; FAUS, M.J. Manual de Atendimento Farmacoterapéutico. Research Group in Pharmaceutical Care, University of Granada, 2004.	

In view of the medicines the patient uses and the health problem identified, a systematic and repetitive process begins which consists of asking three questions for each medicine used or treatments with combinations; and finally, an additional question for the patient's entire pharmacotherapy (Personalized Pharmacotherapy Follow-up).

2.5 *General Anesthetics*

The state of "general anesthesia" usually consists of analgesia, amnesia, loss of consciousness, inhibition of sensory and autonomic reflexes and, in many cases, relaxation of skeletal muscles. The extent to which a given anesthetic drug can exert these effects varies according to the drug, the dose and the clinical circumstances (KATZUNG, 2003).

2.5.1 Inhalation Anesthetics

Nitrous oxide, a gas at room temperature and pressure, remains an important component of many anesthetic regimens. Halothane, enflurane, isoflurane, desflurane, sevoflurane and methoxyflurane are volatile liquids. Older inhalation anesthetics, such as ether, cyclopropane and chloroform, are not used in developed countries for various reasons, including potential flammability (ether, cyclopropane) and organic toxicity (chloroform) (KATZUNG, 2003).

Costa (2002) states that nitrous oxide has moderate analgesic properties, little amnesic action, little immobilizing power and a very mild hypnotic effect. It is therefore understandable that its indications as a single anesthetic agent are very limited, and it is more often used as an adjunct to more powerful inhalational anesthetics in order to reduce their doses and, consequently, their side effects.

Katzung (2003) states that inhalation anesthetics - and most intravenous agents - depress the spontaneous and evoked activity of neurons in many regions of the brain. The original concepts regarding the mechanism of anesthesia suggested the occurrence of nonspecific interactions of these agents with the lipid matrix of the nerve membrane - interactions that were believed to lead to secondary alterations in the flow of ions. The ionic mechanisms involved in the case of different anesthetics may vary; however, at clinically relevant concentrations, they seem to involve interactions with members of the family of channels regulated by fast neurotransmitters. Thus, for example, it has been reported that inhaled anesthetics cause membrane hyperpolarization (an inhibitory action) through the activation of ligand-regulated potassium channels.

In relation to the toxicity of inhaled anesthetics, postoperative liver dysfunction is usually associated with certain factors, such as blood transfusions, hypovolemic shock and other surgical stresses, rather than the toxicity of the anesthetics. However, in a small subgroup of individuals exposed to halothane, the development of potentially serious, life-threatening hepatitis can be seen. Obese patients who have had more than one exposure to halothane over a short period of time may be more susceptible.

The nephrotoxic potential of methoxyflurane has limited its clinical use in anesthesia. Renal dysfunction, which appears after the administration of methoxyflurane, is caused by inorganic fluoride released during the extensive metabolism of the anesthetic by hepatic and renal enzymes. The metabolism of enflurane and sevoflurane also leads to the formation of fluoride ions, raising the question of the potential nephrotoxicity of these anesthetics (KATZUNG, 2003).

2.5.2 Intravenous anesthetics

Various drugs are used intravenously, alone or in combination with other drugs, to produce anesthesia, as components of a balanced anesthetic, or for sedation of patients in intensive care units who need to be mechanically ventilated for prolonged periods of time. Intravenous anesthetics include the following: (1) barbiturates (thiopental, methohexital); (2) benzodiazepines (midazolam, diazepam); (3) opioid analgesics (morphine, fentanyl, sufentanil, alfentanil, remifentanil); (4) propofol; (5) ketamine, an arylcyclohexylamine that produces a state called dissociative anesthesia; (6) other drugs (droperidol, etomidate, dexmedetomidine).

In the last two decades, there has been a growing use of intravenous drugs in anesthesia, both as adjuvants to gaseous anesthetics and in protocols that do not use inhaled anesthetics. Unlike inhaled anesthetics, intravenous agents do not require any specialized equipment for their administration or expensive devices for the recovery and elimination of exhaled gases. Intravenous drugs, such as thiopental, etomidate and propofol, have a faster onset of anesthetic action than even the newer inhalation agents, such as desflurane and sevoflurane. These intravenous agents are commonly used to induce anesthesia. The anesthetic potency of several intravenous agents, including thiopental, ketamine, and propofol, is adequate to allow their use as the sole anesthetic in short-term surgical procedures. Intravenous opioids (e.g. fentanyl) contribute to anesthetic protocols through their cardiovascular stability, sedation and marked analgesia, and opioid receptor antagonists can be used to accelerate the elimination of their actions. Other intravenous agents, such as benzodiazepines (e.g. midazolam, diazepam), are too slow-onset to be of any use as induction agents; however, they can provide a baseline level of sedation for the maintenance of anesthesia when used in association with other agents. Benzodiazepines such as lorazepam and midazolam also provide remarkable anterograde amnesia, a useful action for most patients undergoing anesthesia (KATZUNG, 2003).

Gamma-aminobutyric acid (GABA) and glycine are inhibitory amino acids that act as neurotransmitters in the central nervous system. Three types of GABA receptors have been identified: GABA-A, GABA-B and GABA-C. The GABA-A receptor is part of an ionic complex with chlorine, with muscimol as the agonist and gabazine as the selective antagonist. Barbiturates and alcohol modulate the activity of this receptor by directly facilitating the influx of chlorine. Benzodiazepines bind to a specific site on the GABA-A receptor complex, facilitating GABA-agonist receptor binding and increasing the opening time of the ion channel (ROCHA, 2002).

Although several ultra-short-acting barbiturates are available, thiopental is the most commonly used to induce anesthesia, often in combination with inhalation anesthetics. After intravenous administration, thiopental quickly crosses the blood-brain barrier and, when administered in sufficient doses, produces hypnosis within a short circulation time. Similar effects are observed with other ultra-short-acting barbiturates, such as thiamylal and methohexital. With these barbiturates, equilibrium between the plasma and the brain occurs rapidly (in about a minute), due to their high liposolubility. Thiopental can reduce hepatic blood flow and glomerular filtration rate, but has no lasting effects on liver and kidney function. Barbiturates can exacerbate acute intermittent porphyria by inducing hepatic ALA synthetase. Thiopental has precipitated porphyria crises when used as an inducing agent. Large doses of opioid analgesics have been used to achieve general anesthesia, especially in patients undergoing heart surgery or other major surgery, when circulatory reserve is minimal (KATZUNG, 2003).

Several authors have described that reducing the response to trauma during general anesthesia can be achieved through the use of high doses of intravenous opioids. However, large doses of opioids can cause significant adverse effects and prolong recovery time (NORA, 2007).

The multiple actions exerted by opioids are the result of their interaction with different types of receptors. Studies show that there are several receptors, the most widely accepted being mu (p), kappa, SIGMA, DELTA and EPSILON. The p receptors have been differentiated into two subtypes: p1, with a high affinity for opioids, and p2, with a low affinity. The activities of opioid drugs are manifested according to the interaction and affinity with the receptors and their intrinsic activity (ROCHA, 2002).

Intravenous opioids can increase chest wall rigidity, which can impair ventilation, and postoperative respiratory depression can occur, requiring assisted ventilation and the administration of opioid antagonists, such as naloxone. In addition to its use as a primary anesthetic agent, fentanyl has been used as a premedication and as an adjuvant to inhaled anesthetics. Alfentanil and remifentanil are sometimes used as induction agents, as both drugs have a rapid onset of anesthetic action. Fentanyl and droperidol together produce analgesia and amnesia, and are sometimes used with nitrous oxide to produce neuroleptanesthesia (KATZUNG, 2003).

Half-life, context-dependent, is the time it takes for an agent to decrease its plasma concentration to half of that which was being maintained from the moment its administration was interrupted. It is the parameter most commonly used in intravenous anesthesia to determine the expected time for the end of action of an intravenous drug administered by continuous infusion [1]. Plasma concentrations of sufentanil, fentanyl and alfentanil capable of offering good protection against intraoperative nociceptive stimuli during continuous infusion have context-dependent half-lives ranging from 35 to 45 minutes. Because of this slow recovery profile, associated with the increase in the number of outpatient procedures, as well as the possibility of early extubation in major surgical procedures, remifentanil was introduced. Due to its pharmacokinetic characteristics, remifentanil was developed for continuous administration and has a fast and predictable start and end time (NORA, 2007).

Opioid analgesics are also administered epidurally. Although it cannot prevent the pain caused by the surgical incision, this approach provides profound post-operative analgesia (KATZUNG, 2003).

2,6-diisopropylphenol - propofol or disoprofol - is an extremely important intravenous anesthetic. It produces anesthesia at a similar rate to intravenous barbiturates, and recovery is faster. In particular, patients are able to ambulate sooner after using propofol. In addition, patients "feel better" in the immediate postoperative period after propofol, compared to other intravenous anesthetics. Post-operative vomiting is rare. Propofol has been reported to have antiemetic effects. The drug is also used for both induction and maintenance of anesthesia. It does not appear to cause cumulative effects, nor delayed activation after prolonged infusion. These favorable properties are responsible for the extensive use of propofol as a component of balanced anesthesia and for its great popularity as an anesthetic for use in "day hospital" surgeries. The drug is also effective in producing prolonged sedation in patients in critical care situations. However, the use of propofol for sedation of children in intensive care units has resulted in the development of severe acidosis in the presence of respiratory infections and possible neurological sequelae with its discontinuation.

Etomidate, a carboxylated imidazole, is a powerful hypnotic with no analgesic action. It has similar effects on the central nervous system to barbiturates, acting on the GABAergic system and thus facilitating the inhibitory action of this neurotransmitter (MEDEIROS, 2004). Etomidate is used in the induction of anesthesia, as well as in balanced anesthesia techniques that do not require prolonged administration. Its main advantage over other anesthetics lies in the fact that the drug has minimal cardiovascular and respiratory depressant effects. Etomidate produces loss of consciousness in a matter of seconds, with mild hypotension, no effect on heart rate and a low frequency of apnea. The drug has no analgesic effects, and premedication with opioids may be necessary to decrease cardiac responses during tracheal intubation and reduce spontaneous muscle movements. After an induction dose, recovery occurs within 3 - 5 minutes (KATZUNG, 2003).

Unfortunately, etomidate causes a high incidence of nausea and vomiting, pain after injection, and myoclonus. Involuntary muscle movements are not associated with epileptiform discharges on the EEG. Etomidate can also cause adenocortical pressure through inhibitory effects on steroidogenesis, with a decrease in plasma levels of hydrocortisone after a single dose. Prolonged infusion of etomidate can result in hypotension, electrolyte imbalance and oliguria (KATZUNG, 2003).

Ketamine is a derivative of *phencyclidine hydrochloride* (PCP), synthesized by Stevens in 1965 and its main use is anesthesia in humans and animals (VASCONSELOS, 2005).

Ketamine produces dissociative anaesthesia, characterized by catatonia, amnesia and analgesia, without any real loss of consciousness. The drug is an arylcyclohexylamine chemically related to phencyclidine (PCP), a drug of abuse often used for its psychoactive properties. Ketamine's mechanism of action may involve blocking the effects on the membrane of the excitatory neurotransmitter, glutamic acid, on the NMDA (*N-methyl-D-aspartate*) receptor subtype (KATZUNG, 2003).

Ketamine has been used in humans via the subarachnoid route. Extensive research has been carried out in the past, but has been limited by the drug's potential neurotoxicity. Recent animal studies have failed to demonstrate spinal cord abnormalities following the use of ketamine with preservative. Studies have shown that subarachnoid ketamine increases the analgesic effect of opioids in patients with cancer. Limitations to subarachnoid use include its well-described psychotropic effects and those of vomiting, numbness, arterial hypertension, tachycardia and, rarely, cardiovascular depression (ROCHA, 2002).

Although it is a desirable anesthetic in many respects, ketamine has been associated with disorientation, sensory and perceptual delirium and vivid dreams after anesthesia, effects collectively referred to as "emergence phenomena". Intravenous diazepam, 0.2 - 0.3 mg/kg within five minutes of ketamine administration, reduces the incidence of these phenomena. Due to the high incidence of post-operative psychic phenomena associated with its use, ketamine is not commonly used in general surgery in the United States. It is considered useful for high-risk geriatric patients, as well as for patients in shock, due to its cardiostimulant properties. It is also used in outpatient anesthesia and in changas undergoing painful procedures, such as dressing changes on burned tissue (KATZUNG, 2003).

2.6 *Local anesthetics*

The history of the application of local anesthetics (LA) via the spinal route is quite old, and its use was first documented by Bier in 1899. In 1940, Lemmon introduced the idea of continuous infusion of anesthetic and, in 1948, Lofgren presented his thesis defending the use of spinal lidocaine, which began the application of this substance for surgical procedures (ROCHA, 2002).

Local anesthetics reversibly block the conduction of impulses along the axons of nerves and other excitable membranes that use sodium channels as the main means of generating action potentials. This action can be used clinically to block the sensation of pain coming from specific areas of the body or sympathetic vasoconstrictor impulses directed towards these areas. Cocaine, the first of these drugs, was isolated by Niemann in 1860. It was introduced for clinical use by Koller in 1884 as an ophthalmic anesthetic. It was soon discovered that cocaine had an effect on the central nervous system, causing severe dependence; however, despite this, it was widely used for 30 years and may be the only local anesthetic drug available at the time. In an attempt to improve cocaine's properties, Einhorn synthesized procaine in 1905, which became the dominant local anesthetic for the next 50 years. Since 1905, many local anesthetics have been synthesized. The goals of these efforts were to reduce local irritation and tissue damage, minimize systemic toxicity, achieve a faster onset of action and a longer duration of action. Lidocaine, which remains a popular agent, was synthesized in 1943 by Lofgren and can be considered the prototype of the local anesthetic (KATZUNG, 2003). Lidocaine is often used intravenously during anesthetic induction in order to reduce the hemodynamic responses associated with tracheal intubation (CARDOSO, 2005).

The a2-adrenergic mechanisms of analgesia have been explored for over a hundred years. Cocaine, the first spinal anesthetic, produces analgesia primarily through its action as a local anesthetic, but it also inhibits the reuptake of norepinephrine. The spinal analgesia produced by cocaine is partly due to noradrenergic stimulation of 02 receptors. This discovery prompted the use of 2-adrenergic agonists to achieve analgesia.

However, it wasn't until 1984 that clonidine was successfully administered, when Tamsen et al. [18]after neurotoxicity tests on animals, injected this substance into the epidural spine of two patients with chronic pain. This led to subsequent studies demonstrating the safety of subarachnoid clonidine in the treatment of pain syndromes (ROCHA, 2002).

Local anesthetics such as lidocaine, bupivacaine and, more recently, ropivacaine play a definite role in the management of patients with pain. They act by inactivating voltage-sensitive sodium channels. Their pharmacological action depends on physicochemical characteristics such as molecular weight, liposolubility, degree of ionization and protein affinity. It has been observed that liposolubility determines analgesic potency; pka, the onset of blockade; and protein affinity, the duration of analgesia. Local anesthetics combine with the protein receptor located on the sodium channel of the nerve membrane. Compounds with a higher affinity bind more firmly to the receptor sites, remain in the channel for a longer period of time and have a longer conduction block (ROCHA, 2002).

There is evidence that local anesthetics decrease neuromuscular transmission and exert effects on motor neurons and muscle fibers. *In vitro* studies have shown that the combination of this drug with a neuromuscular blockade results in potentiation of the neuromuscular blocking effects. In clinical practice, this synergistic effect between neuromuscular blockade and local anesthetic could be interesting if it resulted in earlier installation of the neuromuscular blockade, which would enable faster tracheal intubation and protect against the cardiovascular effects inherent in the technique (CARDOSO, 2005).

In general, local anesthetics are administered by injection into the area of the nerve fibers to be blocked. Therefore, absorption and distribution are not as important in controlling the onset of the effect as they are in determining the rate of termination of anesthesia and the likelihood of cardiac and central nervous system toxicity. However, the topical application of local anesthetics requires diffusion of the drug for both the onset and termination of the anesthetic effect (KATZUNG, 2003).

The predominant electrophysiological effect of local anesthetics occurs during the depolarization phase of the action potential. There is a decrease in the speed and degree of depolarization, so that the excitability threshold for transmission is no longer reached and the nerve impulse is no longer propagated along the nerve (ROCHA, 2002).

The primary mechanism of action of local anesthetics - and perhaps the only action in blocking peripheral nerves - consists of voltage-regulated sodium channel blockades. The excitable membrane of nerve axons, like the membrane of cardiac muscle, maintains a transmembrane potential of -90 to - 60 mV. During excitation, the sodium channels open, and a rapid inwardly directed sodium current promptly depolarizes the membrane to the sodium equilibrium potential (+40 mV). As a result of depolarization, the sodium channels close (inactivation), and the potassium channels open. The externally directed flow of potassium repolarizes the membrane to the potassium equilibrium potential (around -95 mV); repolarization causes the sodium channels to return to their resting state. Transmembrane ionic gradients are maintained by the sodium pump. These characteristics are similar to those of the heart muscle, and local anesthetics exert similar effects on both tissues (KATZUNG, 2003).

Local anesthetics are substances which, when in contact with a nerve fiber, have the property of interrupting all modes of nerve flow. When applied to sensitive nerve endings or sensitive nerve trunks, they transiently block the transmission of nerve action potentials, causing loss of sensation (ANTUNES, 2007).

The choice of local anesthetic for a specific procedure is generally based on the duration of action required. Procaine and chloroprocaine are short-acting; lidocaine, mepivacaine and prilocaine are intermediate-acting; and tetracaine, bupivacaine, etidocaine and ropivacaine are long-acting drugs (KATZUNG, 2003).

Bupivacaine (1-butyl-2;6'-pipecolidylxylidase) is widely used in infiltrative anesthesia, as well as in regional blocks. However, its cardiotoxicity and dysrhythmogenic potential mean that it has a narrow safety margin (CANGIANI, 2007).

The effects on the central nervous system at low doses include drowsiness, dazedness, visual and auditory disturbances and restlessness. Even before these effects appear, the patient may notice numbness around the mouth and tongue. At higher concentrations, nystagmus and muscle twitching can occur. Finally, tonic-clonic convulsions can occur, followed by central nervous system depression and death. When applied in excessively high concentrations, all local anesthetics can be toxic to nervous tissue.

The cardiovascular effects of local anesthetics stem partly from direct effects on the cardiac muscle and smooth muscle membrane and partly from indirect effects on the autonomic nerves. Local anesthetics block cardiac sodium channels and therefore depress abnormal cardiac pacemaker activity, excitability and conduction. At very high concentrations, they can also block calcium channels.

The administration of high doses (> 10 mg/kg) of prilocaine during regional anesthesia can lead to an accumulation of the metabolite *o-toluidine,* an oxidizing agent capable of converting hemoglobin into methemoglobin. In the presence of sufficient amounts of methemoglobin (3-5 mg/dL), the patient can become cyanotic, turning the blood a chocolate color. To quickly convert methemoglobin into hemoglobin, reducing agents can be administered intravenously, such as methylene blue or, less satisfactorily, ascorbic acid.

Ester-type local anesthetics are metabolized to p-aminobenzoic acid derivatives. These metabolites are responsible for allergic reactions in a small percentage of the population. Amides are not metabolized to p-aminobenzoic acid, and allergic reactions to drugs in the amine group are extremely rare (KATZUNG, 2003).

Chapter 3
3. METHODOLOGY

3.1 Characterizing the Universe:

The study was carried out in a public hospital in the city of Campiña Grande - PB, the FAP hospital, through a qualitative-quantitative approach, through descriptive and exploratory research, using a cross-sectional and descriptive study, which focused on the consumption of anaesthetics by hospitalized patients undergoing pharmacological treatment with anaesthetic drugs.

The Fundagao Assistencial da Paraíba, the FAP Hospital, operates with 200 beds, 150 of which are for medical and surgical clinics and 50 beds for the Dr. Ulisses Pinto Cancer Center.

3.2 Characterizing the Sample:

The sample was made up of patients admitted to the hospital who had undergone the use of anesthetics during the period of this study. The research will be carried out from August 2007 to July 2008. Patients of both sexes were included, regardless of age, color or social class, who were admitted to the surgical ward.

3.3 Data Collection Instrument:

A standard questionnaire specifically designed for the study was used as a data collection tool. This questionnaire is a simple and objective instrument which contains basic information on patient identification, use of medication, use of other associated medication, treatment progress and detection of possible adverse reactions. It was filled in by analyzing medical records and observing hospitalized patients (Appendix 01).

3.4 *Data Analysis:*

The data was analyzed using Windows Excel 2003. The data collected was entered into tables and figures so that a quantitative analysis could be carried out, taking into account the relative and absolute values that justify the prevalence of responses.

Once the results were in, a qualitative approach was taken, comparing the data obtained with the scientific literature.

3.5 *Ethical considerations:*

The project was submitted to UEPB's ethics committee and was approved in accordance with Resolution 196/96 of the National Health Council. The patients were informed in advance about the aims of the study, and were guaranteed the right to withdraw from taking part in the research, as well as the confidentiality of the information collected, safeguarding their right to privacy, and there was no need to identify them. Everyone signed a free and informed consent form during the research.

Chapter 4

4. RESULTS

During the study period, 65 patients who used anesthetics were analyzed. There was a prevalence of females (Figure 01). The data was grouped into four age groups. The ages ranged from twenty to eighty-one. The age group with the highest prevalence of anesthetic use was between 41 and 60 years (Figure 02).

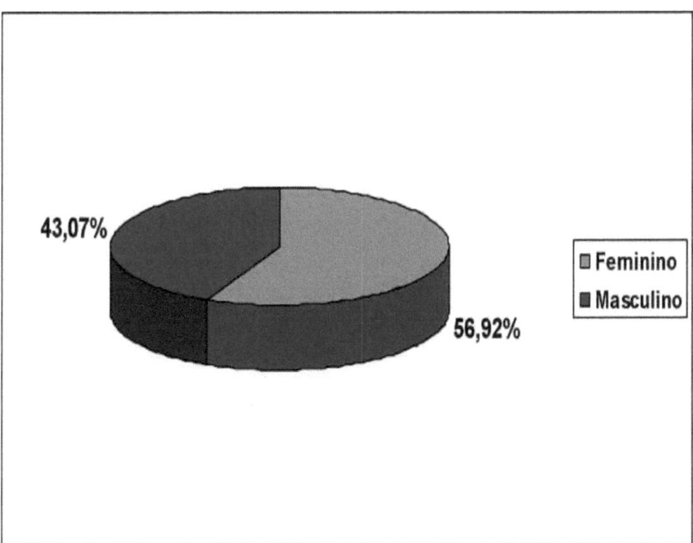

Figure 1 - Percentage distribution of the patients studied according to gender.

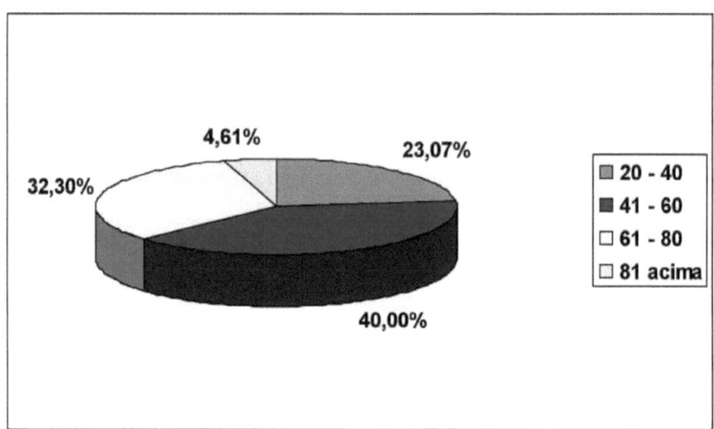

Figure 02 - Percentage distribution of patients analyzed by age group.

Figure 03 shows the surgical procedures the patients underwent. Of all the patients interviewed, hysterectomy accounted for a significant percentage of the total.

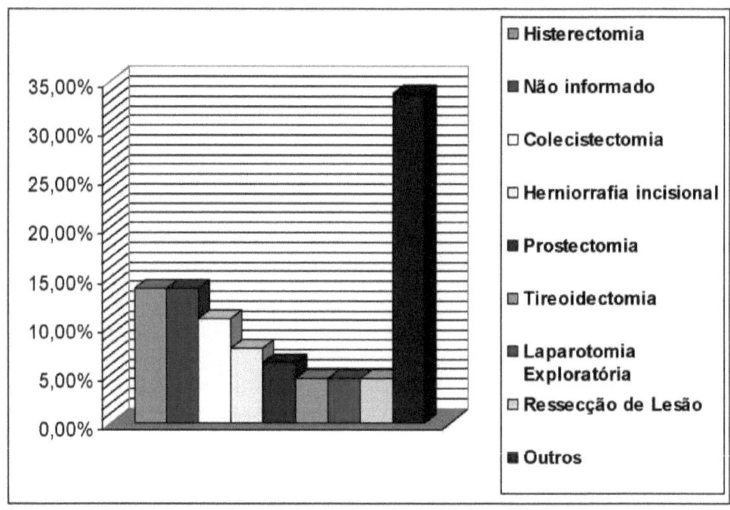

Figure 03 - Percentage distribution of surgical procedures recorded in

patients' medical records, which used anesthetics.

Figure 04 shows the incidence of hypertension among the patients interviewed.

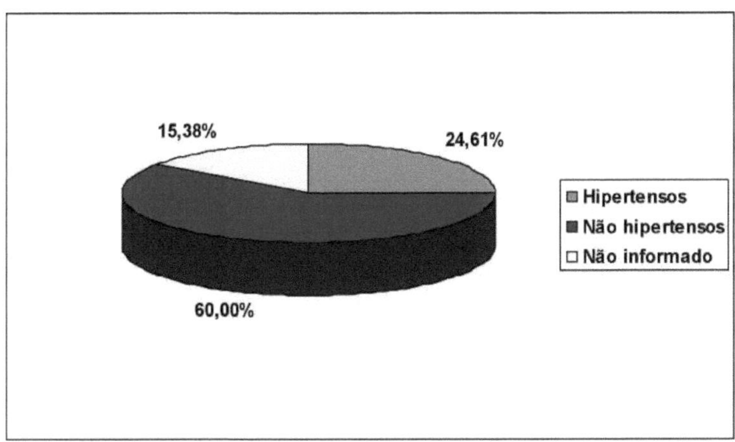

Figure 04 - Percentage distribution of the incidence of hypertension among the

patients interviewed.

Among the anesthetics studied, heavy bupivacaine had the highest incidence in

the study, followed by morphine and midazolam, as shown in Figure 05.

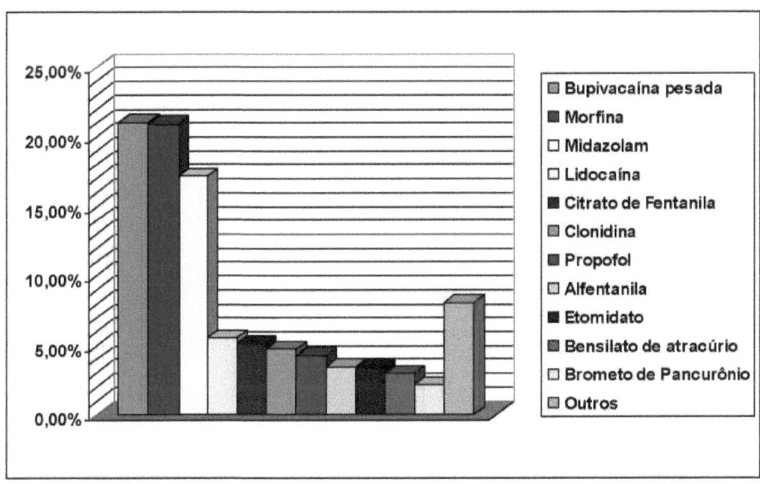

Figure 05 - Percentage distribution of the types of anesthetics used by the

patients analyzed.

It was observed that the majority of patients had possible adverse drug reactions (ADRs), as shown in Figure 06.

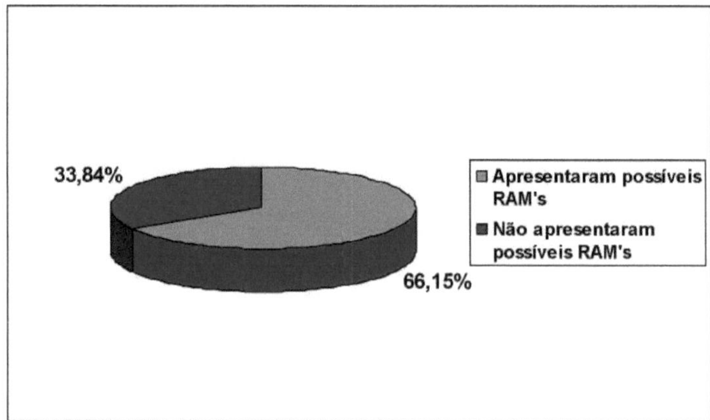

Figure 06 - Percentage distribution of patients in terms of

possible ADRs.

Figure 07 shows the possible ADRs caused by the use of anesthetics in the patients analyzed.

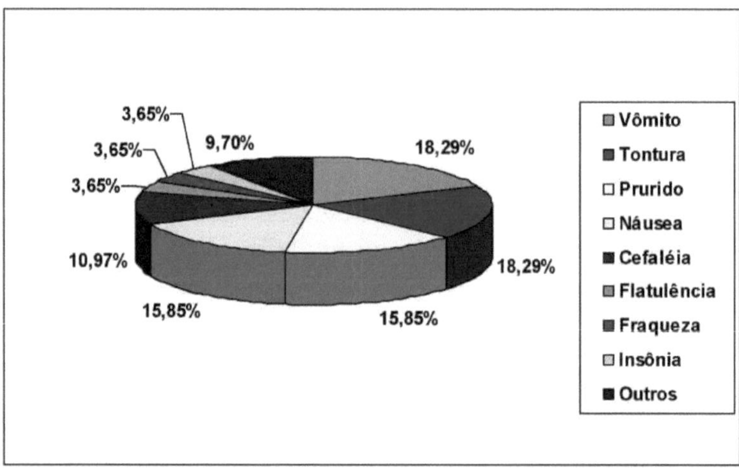

Figure 07 - Percentage distribution of possible adverse reactions to medication

caused by the use of anesthetics.

The drugs used concomitantly during the surgical procedure were analyzed, as shown in Figure 08.

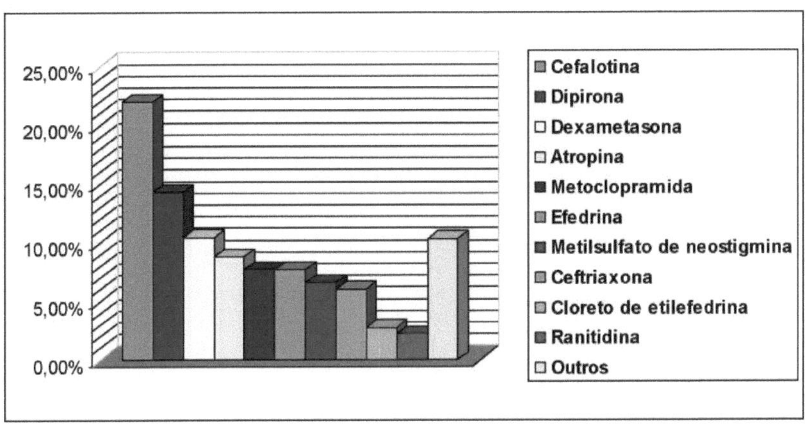

Figure 08 - Percentage distribution of the prevalence of concomitant use of medication during the surgical procedure.

Figure 09 shows the prevalence of medications used by patients in the post-surgical period.

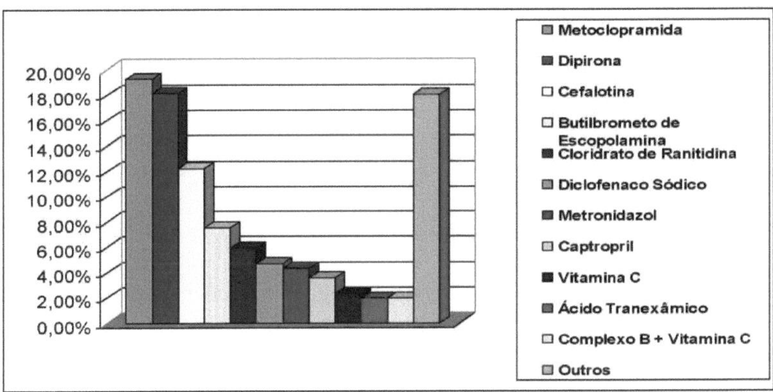

Figure 09 - Percentage distribution of the prevalence of medicines used by patients in the post-surgical period.

Chapter 5

5. DISCUSSION

The results of this study draw attention to the prevalence of women among the patients analyzed, since women are more susceptible to adverse reactions, possibly due to an association of factors. It is also possible that there is a hormonal determinant that can affect metabolism, predisposing the appearance of adverse reactions (GOMES, 2001).

In terms of age group, there was a prevalence between 41 and 60 years, which shows that the majority of the patients analyzed were non-elderly.

Hysterectomy was the surgical procedure with the highest incidence during the study. According to Costa *et al* (2003), hysterectomy is one of the most frequently performed gynecological surgeries in hospitals around the world. The most frequent indications are benign diseases (uterine leiomyomatosis, endometriosis, hyperplasia), while malignant diseases account for around 10% of indications.

Although the results show that there was no prevalence of hypertension among patients who used anesthetic drugs, it is worth highlighting the importance of hypertension in relation to the use of anesthetics. According to Lorentz *et al* (2005), the appropriate control of blood pressure in the preoperative period, as well as the approach to hypertensive patients by anesthesiologists, has been the subject of constant debate over the last 30 years. According to the same author, in a large study carried out with patients who were candidates for orthopaedic surgery, hypertension was the main medical cause of surgery suspensions, accounting for 16.2% of cases. Lorentz (2005) also mentions that it has already been established that poorly controlled hypertensive patients generally present more intense hemodynamic alterations during surgery; there is a pronounced and relatively greater decrease in blood pressure after induction of anesthesia and, generally, **an** increased response to the stress of intubation and extubation.

Among the patients analyzed, most had possible adverse drug reactions. The most commonly reported possible ADRs were vomiting and dizziness, followed by nausea and pruritus. According to Santos *et al* (2006), in general, the adverse effects reported in the immediate postoperative period of minor surgery are nausea and vomiting, bleeding, pain, headache and fever. In this author's study, the most frequent adverse effects were vomiting and nausea, followed by moderate or severe pain.

Heavy bupivacaine was the most commonly used anesthetic during the study, followed by morphine and midazolam. According to Cangiani *et al* (2007), bupivacaine (1-butyl-2;6'-pipecolidylxylidase) is widely used in infiltrative anesthesia, as well as in regional blocks. However, its cardiotoxicity and dysrhythmogenic potential mean that it has a narrow safety margin. In relation to morphine, Torres Neto *et al* (2007) cites that the efficacy of morphine derivatives associated with local anesthetics has traditionally been proven in obtaining good post-operative analgesia when performing spinal or epidural anesthesia. In relation to midazolam, Katzung (2003) states that intravenous agents such as benzodiazepines (e.g. midazolam, diazepam) are too slow-onset to be of any use as induction agents; however, they can provide a baseline level of sedation for the maintenance of anesthesia when used in association with other agents. Benzodiazepines, such as lorazepam and midazolam, also provide remarkable anterograde amnesia, a useful action for most patients undergoing anesthesia.

Among the drugs used concomitantly during the surgical procedure, cephalothin had the highest percentage. Costa (2004) considers that post-surgical infection is a major health problem and mentions that in the United States, it is estimated that of the 23 million surgeries performed each year, 920,000 are complicated by surgical wound infections, which is associated with increased hospitalization time, lethality rates and hospital costs. According to the Ministry of Health guidelines (1998) on antibiotic prophylaxis in surgery, the use of antimicrobials can prevent the occurrence of post-operative infection at the surgical site in various types of surgery, including hysterectomies. However, information and references regarding the examination of the corresponding scientific evidence are not mentioned in the document.

CONCLUSIONS

It can therefore be concluded that the majority of the patients analyzed were female, aged between 41 and 60. With regard to the surgical procedures the patients underwent, hysterectomy had the highest percentage and most of the patients were not hypertensive. Among the anesthetics studied, heavy bupivacaine was the most common, followed by morphine and midazolam. It was also observed that the majority of patients had possible Adverse Drug Reactions (ADRs), of which vomiting and dizziness accounted for the highest percentage, followed by pruritus and nausea. The drugs used concomitantly during the surgical procedure were analyzed, of which cephalothin and dipyrone had the highest percentage. In the post-surgical period, the most commonly used drugs were metoclopramide, followed by dipyrone and cephalothin.

The results of this study serve as a basis for future studies on the choice of appropriate anesthetic techniques for surgical procedures, with the aim of minimizing the occurrence of adverse effects that could prolong hospitalization. This is expected to reduce hospital costs, free up beds for cases of greater need, reduce hospitalization time and reduce the risk of hospital infection.

REFERENCES

ANTUNES et al. Knowledge of FOP/UPE undergraduate students regarding local anesthetic dosage. **Rev. Cir. Traumatol.** Camaragibe v.7, n.1, p. 71 - 78, jan./mar. 2007.

ANVISA. **News**. Available at <http://www.anvisa.gov.br/divulga/noticias/2004/0605042.htm> Accessed on August 16, 2004.

CANGIANI, L.; CANGIANI, L.; PEREIRA, A. M.de S. A. Bupivacaine with enantiomeric excess (S75-R25) at 0.5%, racemic bupivacaine at 0.5% and lidocaine at 2% in facial nerve block using the O'Brien technique: a comparative study. **Rev. Bras. Anestesiol.**, Campinas, v. 57, n. 2, 2007.

CARDOSO, L. S. M.; MARTINS, C. R.; TARDELLI, M. A. Effects of intravenous lidocaine on the pharmacodynamics of rocuronium. **Rev. Bras. Anestesiol.**, Campinas, v. 55, n. 4, 2005.

CASTRO, L. L. C. de. Pharmacoepidemiology in Brazil: evolution and perspectives.
Cienc. saúde coletiva, Rio de Janeiro, v. 4, n. 2,   1999.

CASTRO, L. L. C. de. Fundamentals of Pharmacoepidemiology. Campo Grande: Rational Use of Medicines Research Group **GRUPURAM**, 2001.

CICARELLI, D. D. et al. Importance of training residents in adverse events during anesthesia: experience with the use of a computerized simulator. **Rev. Bras. Anestesiol.**, Campinas, v. 55, n. 2, 2005.

COELHO, H. L. Pharmacovigilance: a necessary tool. **Cad. Saúde Pública**, Rio de Janeiro, 14(4):871-875, Oct-Dec, 1998.
COELHO, H. L.; ARRAIS, P. S. D. Development of pharmacoepidemiology in Brazil: I Seminário Brasileiro de

Farmacoepidemiologia. **Cad. Saúde Pública**. Rio de Janeiro, v. 15, n. 1, 1999.

COSTA, A. A. R.; AMORIM, M .M. R. de; CURSINO, T. Vaginal hysterectomy versus abdominal hysterectomy in women without genital prolapse, in a maternity school in Recife: a randomized clinical trial. **Rev. Bras. Ginecol. Obstet.**, Apr. 2003, vol.25, no.3, p.169-176.

COSTA, RJM; KRAUSS-SILVA, L. Systematic review and meta-analysis of antibiotic prophylaxis in abdominal hysterectomy. **Cad. Saúde Pública**. Rio de Janeiro, 20 Sup 2:S175-S189, 2004.

COSTA, V. V. da; SARAIVA, R. A. Action of nitrous oxide on the central nervous system: electrophysiological study as a single agent and as an adjuvant agent. **Rev. Bras. Anestesiol.**, Campinas, v. 52, n. 3, 2002.

EINARSON, TR. Drug-related hospital admissions. **Ann Pharmacother** 1993; 27: 832-40.

GOMES, M. J. V. de M.; REIS, A. M. M.. **Pharmaceutical Sciences: a hospital pharmacy approach**. 1st edition. Sao Paulo: Atheneu Publishing House, 2001.

HALLAS, J; GRAM, LF;GRODUM, E; DAMSBO, N; BROSEN, K; HAGHFELT, T; et al. Drug related admissions to medical wards: a population based study. **Br J Clin Pharmacol** 1992; 33:61-8.

KATZUNG, B. G. **Basic and Clinical Pharmacology**. 8ª . Edigao. Guanabara Koogan: Rio de Janeiro, 2003.

LORENTZ, M. N.; SANTOS, A. X. Systemic arterial hypertension and anesthesia. **Rev. Bras. Anestesiol.**, Campinas, v. 55, n. 5, 2005.

MACHUCA, M; FERNÁNDEZ-LLIMÓS, F; FAUS, M.J. Manual de Atención Farmacoterapéutico. Pharmaceutical Care Research Group, **University of Granada,** 2004.

MEDEIROS, C. G. S., et al. Comparative analysis of the effects of diazepam, midazolam, propofol and etomidate on myocardial contractility and coronary flow: study in isolated rat hearts. **Rev Bras Cir Cardiovasc**, 19(2): 157-164, 2004.

MINISTRY OF HEALTH. Coordination of Hospital Infection Control. Consensus on the rational use of antimicrobials. Brasilia: Coordination of Hospital Infection Control, **Ministry of Health**; 1998.

NISHIYAMA, P.; BONETTI, M. de F. de S.; BOHM, A. C. F.; MARGONATO, F. B.. Pharmacovigilance Experience at the Regional University Hospital of Maringá, State of Paraná. **Maringá**, v. 24, n. 3, p. 749-755, 2002.

NORA, F. S. et al. Remifentanil: does the infusion regimen make a difference in preventing circulatory responses to tracheal intubation? **Rev. Bras. Anestesiol.**, Campinas, v. 57, n. 3, 2007.

WORLD HEALTH ORGANIZATION. The selection of essential medicines. Geneva, **WHO,** 1977.

PFAFFENBACH, G.; CARVALHO, O. M.; MENDES, G. B. Adverse Drug Reactions as Determinants of Hospital Admission. **Rev. Assoc. Med. Bras**. v.48 n.3 Sao Paulo jul./set. 2002.

PRANDO, L. E.; SILVA, D. D. The Difficulties of Professional Pharmacists in Implementing Pharmaceutical Care and Pharmacovigilance in Hospital and Community Pharmacies. **Infarma**, v.16, n° 11-12, 2004.

ROCHA, Anita Perpétua Carvalho; LEMONICA, Lino; BARROS, Guilherme Antônio
Moreira de. Use of subarachnoid medication in the treatment of chronic pain.
Rev. Bras. Anestesiol., Campinas, v. 52, n. 5, 2002.
SANTOS, A. C. P. et al. Adverse effects in the postoperative period of surgery
gynecological and breast diseases. **Rev. Assoc. Med. Bras.**, Sao Paulo, v. 52, n. 4, 2006.

TORRES NETO, J. da R. et al. Evaluation of postoperative analgesia in patients undergoing orificial surgery with local anesthesia associated or not with morphine. Rev bras. colo-proctol., Rio de Janeiro, v. 27, n. 1, 2007.

VASCONCELOS, S. M. M. et al. Ketamine: general aspects and relationship with schizophrenia. **Rev. psiquiatr. clín.**, Sao Paulo, v. 32, n. 1, 2005.

WORLD HEALTH ORGANIZATION - WHO. International drug monitoring: the role of the hospital. Report of a WHO meeting. Geneva: **WHO**; 1969. p.1-24.

Appendix

<table>
<tr>
<td rowspan="2">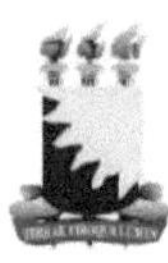</td>
<td>**STATE UNIVERSITY OF PARAÍBA**

ASSISTANCE FOUNDATION OF PARAÍBA

PHARMACOVIGILANCE SECTOR</td>
<td>File no:

Date:</td>
</tr>
</table>

1. PERSONAL DATA:

Proceedings: ____

Age:Profession:

Weight: ____________ Sex: ( )M ()   F

Date of admission: __________________

Date of departure: __________________

2.0 INSTITUTIONAL DATA:

Sector: (   ) Ward   () Apartment   (   )

Outpatient: ______________________________________

Patient follow-up begins: ________________________________

End of patient follow-up: ________________________________

30 CLINICAL DATA:

Clinical History ______________________________________

Pathology: ______________________________________

Symptoms: ______________________________________

Surgery: ______________________________________

Date of diagnosis: _____ / __ / _____   Date of surgery : __ / ___ / __

Other existing pathologies (chronic degenerative): ______________

Allergy to medication: (   ) Yes   (   ) No

Which one(s): ____

Patient complaints during treatment: ____________________________

Data from clinical-laboratory examinations: ____________________

Do you use any special diet? (   ) Yes   (   ) No

Which one(s): ____

4.0 PHARMACOVIGILANCE

- Anesthetics used in the hospital during the hospitalization period, which

(is)? ____

- Dosage: ____

Others: ____

- Did you use medication before your hospitalization?( ) Yes (   ) No

Which one(s): ____

Prescribed by a doctor? ( ) Yes   () No

- Have there been any adverse reactions to the drug since it was administered?

( ) Yes   () No

Which one(s): ____

If Positive:

- Have you discontinued the medication? (   ) Yes (   ) No

- Was it administered again? (   ) Yes   (   ) No

- Have you noticed any new adverse reactions?

( ) Yes (   ) No

Which one(s): ____

- Have you been given any other medication? (   ) Yes (   ) No

Which one(s): ____

____

- Have there been any adverse reactions to the new medication administered?

( ) Yes   () No

Which one(s)______________________________   :

____

____

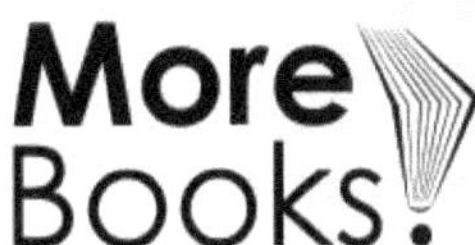

More
Books!

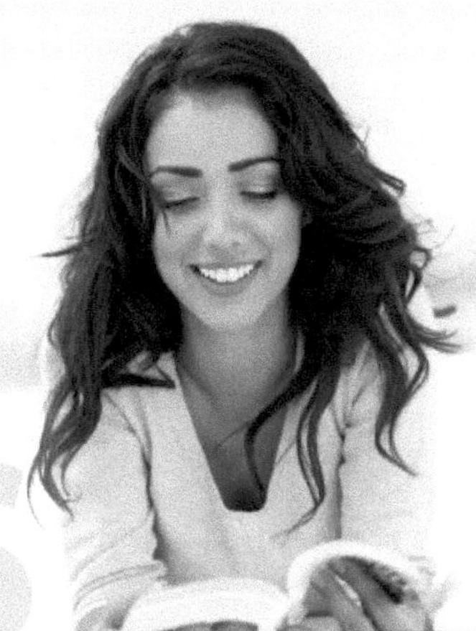

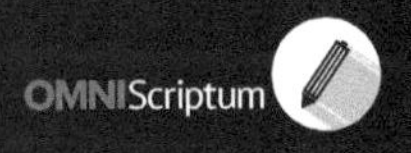

info@omniscriptum.com
www.omniscriptum.com
OMNIScriptum

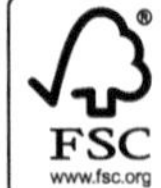